Ketogenic Miracle

Enhancing Health while Increasing Weight Loss Success
How can you avoid Ketogenic Diet mistakes

By: *Emily Simmons*

Disclaimer:

The information presented in this book represents the views of the publisher as of the date of publication. The publisher reserves the rights to alter update their opinions based on new conditions. This report is for informational purposes only. The author and the publisher do not accept any responsibilities for any liabilities resulting from the use of this information. While every attempt has been made to verify the information provided here, the author and the publisher cannot assume any responsibility for errors, inaccuracies or omissions. Any similarities with people or facts are unintentional.

Table of Contents

Chapter 1 7
    What is the Ketogenic Diet? 7

Chapter 2 9
    What should you eat? 9

Chapter 3 15
    What Can You Expect From the Ketogenic Diet? 15

Chapter 4 19
    What, apart from willpower, is needed to start the Ketogenic Diet? 19
        How to get started 19

Chapter 5 25
Chapter 6 37
    How can you avoid Ketogenic Diet mistakes? 37

Conclusion 41

Introduction

Folks, you have this amazing book called ***Ketogenic Diet Mistakes You Need to Know*** in your hands. You must have already read a lot about the Ketogenic Diet before starting it. Of course, it is always easy to start something, but a lot more difficult to stick to it. This doesn't only apply to difficult things. Many people struggle to see even a small commitment through to the end.

A lot more than determination and willpower are needed to stay committed to the Ketogenic Diet. This book deals with the requirements and hazards of the Ketogenic Diet in full detail. Go through the chapters given in this book. You will not find any dearth of knowledge about this "intimidating" diet. You will hopefully feel more enlightened after reading this book, because it sheds enough light on the concept to chase away all your feelings of intimidation. Before just jumping into the area that deals with common mistakes, we have given you some general information on the Ketogenic Diet- the foods you should and shouldn't eat, things you must and must not do, and the possible mistakes that you need to learn to watch out for. It is smarter to learn from the mistakes of others. It saves you much time, energy, and money. Otherwise, when you do not take the precautionary steps and keep making the mistakes, you'll quickly start to feel miserable and will most likely quit the regime.

You have made a smart move by starting with this book. This proves that you are willing to improve your well-being. We have very fast lives these days and it is always better to be prepared beforehand rather than repent later. If you have already started the Ketogenic regime, you still have enough time to learn the hazards in case you have been unintentionally causing trouble for yourself. If you have not yet started it, please take the time to read this Bible of the Ketogenic Diet and only then take your first step. We'll lay any lingering anxieties you may have to rest. Why not invite a few friends along on this health-filled journey and ask them to support you if they are willing? It's always easier to complete the course when you have someone along with you.

Just set aside your inhibitions and let's get started.
Remember to enjoy the journey rather than only look at the target.
Our best wishes are with you!

Chapter 1

What is the Ketogenic Diet?

The Ketogenic Diet, also known as Keto Diet, is based on the concept of eating fewer carbohydrates and more fats. This makes the body produce ketones in the liver that are used as energy. You must be wondering what ketones are. Well, they are the acids or organic compounds which are produced when our bodies start using fats for energy in place of carbohydrates. When our bodies do not have enough glucose obtained from sugar in the blood to transport it into the cells, our bodies use fats instead and break them down to supply us with energy. However, high levels of ketones are harmful for the body, and may lead to a condition called ketoacidosis.

The Ketogenic Diet has been in existence for more than 5 decades, but has risen in popularity in the last few years. It is famously known by many names: Low Carbs Diet, LCHF (Low Carb High Fat Diet), Keto Diet, etc.

When our diets are rich in carbohydrates, our body produces insulin and glucose.

It is easiest for the body to make energy from glucose. Thus, it automatically chooses glucose over any other molecule to convert it into energy. Insulin performs the activity of taking glucose around your body and processes it in your bloodstream. Now, you can understand that since glucose is mainly used as a primary source of energy, fats are not usually used and therefore they are stored in different parts of our bodies. This makes our bodies bulky.

Our normal diet is high in carbohydrates, which provides glucose as the primary source of energy. When we lower the intake of carbohydrates, the body is encouraged to enter into a condition called ketosis. It is a natural process, which is initiated by the body when we consume less food. During this condition, our body produces ketones by breaking down fats taken from the liver.

The primary goal of a well maintained ketogenic diet is to encourage our bodies to enter this state of metabolism. This does not mean that we have to starve for calories, but we do need to cut down on carbohydrates. This has a plus side to it. We can indulge in a lot of fats and still not feel guilty about it. However, we need to look out for some common mistakes, which we will talk about later.

Our bodies are made to be extremely adaptive. We can put them through whatever conditions we have to and they can adjust. Even when we snatch a major portion of carbohydrates from our diet, we will not feel weak once our bodies adapt to the new diet. They will start utilizing ketones as the primary source of energy.

Chapter 2

What should you eat?

If you want to begin the Ketogenic Diet, you will need to plan very well because this diet does not suit everyone. You must have a practicable diet plan before you begin. Whatever you consume depends on how quickly you want to enter into the state of ketosis. The faster you quit carbohydrates, the quicker you will reach ketosis. Normally, the net amount of carbs specified for the Keto Diet is 20-30 grams every day. You might be wondering, "What are net carbs?" Don't worry. It's really simple. "Net carbs" means the total carbs in your diet minus the amount of fiber. For example, 100 grams of lettuce contains 3 grams of carbohydrates and 1.3 grams of dietary fiber. So, we can deduce that if we subtract 1.3 grams of fiber from 3 grams of carbohydrates, we are left with 1.7 grams of net carbs.

It may be a challenge to stick to a healthy diet low on carbs, particularly when you have just started it. However, owing to the popularity of this diet nowadays, you will not find any shortage of recipes to look for which contain fewer carbohydrates. You can go through the list below of foods friendly to the Keto Diet to help you make the appropriate choices. You must keep one thing in mind: that you have to eat real food, not only food that is low in carbohydrates.

Foods like eggs, meats, nuts, vegetables, yoghurt, and some fruits occasionally. Also, you must avoid any kind of processed food which may contain colorings and preservatives.

Following the Ketogenic Diet does not mean that you have to lose weight regardless of the cost. It is all about taking on a healthier lifestyle.

You can eat these things freely:
Wild animals and grass fed animal sources of protein

Grass fed meat simply means that it is the meat of an animal which grazes grass. You can indulge in the grass fed meat of goat, lamb, beef, and venison.

Wild caught seafood and fish, pastured poultry and pork, ghee, gelatin, pastured eggs, and butter. These foods have a high content of omega 3 fatty acids.

You must keep away from farmed fish, meat and sausages covered with breadcrumbs, meat which comes with starchy or sugary sauces, and hot dogs.

You can also eat the offal (heart, liver, kidneys, and meat of other organs) of grass fed animals.

Healthy fats

Saturated fats like tallow, lard, goose fat, duck fat, clarified butter or ghee, coconut oil, butter.

Monounsaturated fat like macadamia, avocado, olive oil.

Polyunsaturated omega 3's, from animal sources like seafood and fatty fish.

Non-starchy vegetables

Cruciferous vegetables like kohlrabi, kale, and radish leaves.

Leafy greens like bok choy, Swiss chard, lettuce, spinach, endive, chives, radicchio, etc.

Celery stalks, cucumber, asparagus, summer squash (spaghetti squash, zucchini), bamboo shoots.

Condiments and beverages

Coffee (with coconut cream or black coffee), still water, black or herbal tea.

Pork rinds for breading.

Mustard, mayonnaise, homemade bone broth, pesto, pickles, homemade fermented foods like kombucha, kimchi, sauerkraut, etc.

All herbs and spices, lime or lemon zest and juice.

Whey protein, egg white protein, grass fed and hormone free gelatin.

Keep away from artificial sweeteners, additives, soy lecithin, hormones.

Fruits

Avocado

You can eat these foods occasionally:

Fruits, vegetables and mushrooms

Cruciferous vegetables like green and white cabbage, cauliflower, red cabbage, broccoli, fennel, Brussels sprouts, turnips, swede/ rutabaga.

Nightshades (eggplant, peppers, tomatoes).

Root vegetables like parsley root, leek, spring onion, onion, mushrooms, garlic, winter squash like pumpkin.

Sea vegetables like kombu, and nori; okra, bean sprouts, wax beans,

sugar snap peas, water chestnuts, globe or French artichokes.
Berries (blueberries, blackberries, strawberries, cranberries, raspberries, mulberries, etc.)
Coconut, rhubarb, olives.

Full-fat dairy and grain-fed animals

Beef, eggs, poultry, and ghee (stay away from farmed pork, as it has high content of omega 6's!)

Dairy products (cottage cheese, full-fat yogurt, sour cream, cream, cheese.)

Stay away from products which are labeled "low-fat". Many of these products are packed with starch and sugar. They do not have any satiating effect.

Bacon. Be cautious of added starches and preservatives. You can consume nitrates if you have antioxidants in your diet.

Seeds and nuts

Macadamia nuts which are low in carbs and high in omega 3's.
Almonds, pecans, walnuts, pine nuts, hazelnuts, flaxseed, sesame seeds, sunflower seeds, hemp seeds, pumpkin seeds.
Brazil nuts (be cautious of their high selenium content, and eat only very small amount of them.

Soy products (fermented)

If you eat any soy products, eat only fermented or non GMO soy products like tempeh, natto, soy sauce or coconut aminos (paleo-friendly).
Green soy beans or edamame, unprocessed black soy beans.

Condiments

Zero carbohydrate healthy sweeteners (Swerve, Stevia, Erythritol, etc.)
Tomato products (sugar free) like passata, puree, ketchup.
Thickeners like xanthan gum, and arrowroot powder. Remember that xanthan gum is not a paleo friendly gum; still it is used by many paleo followers since you need only a small amount of it.
Extra dark chocolate (it is better to take 70% or 90% chocolate, do not take any soy lecithin), carob and cocoa powder.
Do not take mints and chewing gums. Some of them contain carbohydrates.

Some fruits, vegetables, seeds and nuts with limited

carbohydrates- depending on your daily limit of carbohydrates

- Root vegetables (carrot, celery root, beetroot, sweet potato, and parsnip)
- Watermelon Cantaloupe / Honeydew melons/ Galia
- Cashew and pistachio nuts, chestnuts
- Very small amounts of dragon fruits, apricots, peaches, apples, nectarines, grapefruits, kiwi berries, kiwifruit, oranges, cherries, plums, figs (fresh), pears

Alcohol

You can drink dry white wine, dry red wine, or unsweetened spirits. However, if you are on a weight loss regime, it is best to avoid them. These drinks should only be taken once you reach the weight maintenance stage.

You must avoid these foods:

It is important to avoid food containing a high content of carbohydrates, processed foods and factory farmed meat.

All kinds of grains and artificial sweets

Avoid whole grains such as wheat, oats, corn, rye, barley, bulgur, sorghum, millet, rice, amaranth, sprouted grains, and buckwheat. This automatically encompasses products made of grains like pasta, pizza, bread, crackers, cookies, etc.

Avoid white potatoes and quinoa

Avoid sugar, sweets, etc. like table sugar, agave syrup, HFCS, ice-creams, sweet puddings, cakes, and sugary soft-drinks

Fish and pork farmed in factories

They have high content of omega 6 fatty acids which causes inflammation in the body. Farmed fish also contains PCBs. You must also avoid fish with a high mercury content.

Artificial sweeteners

Splenda, sweeteners containing Aspartame, Equal, Acesulfame, Saccharin, Sucralose, etc.

Processed foods

Processed foods which contain carrageenan
MSG (it is contained in a few whey protein products
Sulphites in gelatin and dried fruits
BPAs, they are not always labeled
Wheat gluten

Refined oils and fats
Sunflower, safflower, canola, cottonseed, soybean, corn oil, grapeseed
Trans-fats such as margarine

Products labeled low fat, low carbs, zero carbs
Atkins products, diet drinks and soda
Chewing mints and gums may contain a high content of carbs, or they may also contain gluten, artificial additives, etc.

Milk
A very small amount of full fat raw milk is permissible on the Ketogenic Diet.
Other than that, milk is prohibited for many reasons. Among all dairy products, milk is the most difficult one to digest because it contains few good bacteria. (They are destroyed during pasteurization.) Milk may also contain hormones.
Also, milk is high in carbohydrates. There are almost 4-5 grams of carbs in 100 milliliters of milk.
If you want to make tea or coffee, you can put cream in measured amounts.
Though you can drink small quantities of milk, you must make a note of the total carbohydrates.

Sweet drinks and alcohol
Sweet wine, beer, and cocktails must be avoided.

Tropical fruits
Mango, pineapple, papaya, and banana should be avoided.
Fruits high in carbs should also be avoided such as grapes, tangerines, etc.
You must also avoid fruit juices (both packed and fresh). However, you may drink smoothies in limited quantities. Juices are like water with sugar, but smoothies contain fiber, and they are more satiating.

You must also avoid large quantities of dried fruits like raisins and dates. You may consume them in moderate quantities.

Soy products

You must avoid most of the soy products, excluding non-GMO fermented products that are good for health.

Other things to keep away from

You must keep away from wheat gluten which is present in low-carbs foods. You will have to give up bread.

Stay away from cans lined with BPA. If possible, you must look for BPA-free containers like glass jars. BPA is partly responsible for many health ailments like impaired thyroid function, cancer, etc.

[BPA implies bisphenol A. It is a chemical used in industries which make a particular kind of resins and plastics. It is normally found in epoxy resins and polycarbonate plastics. Such plastics are used to make containers that store beverages and food. Epoxy resins are applied on the inside of containers like food cans, water supply lines and bottle tops.

Research has shown that BPA is capable of seeping into beverages and foods from these containers, which is terrible for health. Thus, it is better to avoid products packed in such containers.]

You must avoid other additives like carrageenan, MSG, sulfites.

Chapter 3

What Can You Expect From the Ketogenic Diet?

Benefits of following the Ketogenic Diet:

What benefits do you get from following such a strict diet? There are many. Not only does the Ketogenic Diet help you to lose weight, but it also gives you the following advantages:

Cholesterol: The Ketogenic Diet improves your cholesterol and triglyceride levels, which are mostly linked with the clogging up of arteries.
Weight loss: Since your body burns fat for energy in this diet, your body weight automatically comes down during the state of fasting.
Blood sugar: LDL cholesterol decreases over time with the Keto diet;
The symptoms of type 2 diabetes can be controlled over time with the Keto diet
Energy: Fats are more effective and long lasting source molecules to be burned as fuel by our bodies. Since they are a more dependable source of energy, you should feel even more energized on the Ketogenic Diet.
Hunger: Fats keep us satiated for longer hours and we feel hungry less often. Obviously, when we consume less, we gain less weight.
Acne: On a keto diet, you can recognize a drop in skin inflammation and acne lesions in just 12 weeks.

Why physical performance goes down temporarily on a ketogenic diet:

When you begin any new diet, your body needs time to adapt to it. This is also the case with the Ketogenic Diet. When you first start eating food high in fats and low in carbohydrates, you may see some limitations to the physical performance of your body. However, as soon as your body completely adapts to using fats as the main source of energy, you will start to regain your endurance and strength very quickly.

Many people are curious about whether they need carbohydrates to build strength and muscles. Absolutely not. When you work out to make muscles, you need to understand how your body processes food to gain mass and strengthen up well. Protein is the key.

Your body storage of glycogen can be refilled when you are on the Ketogenic Diet. This diet allows you to build good muscles, but there is a trick. You have to keep a check on your protein intake. Experts suggest that you must take in between 1.0-1.2 grams of protein for each lean pound of your body mass. You might find it difficult to gain mass on the Ketogenic Diet because the total fat in your body does not increase on the Ketogenic Diet. If for any reason you want to put on weight, you can do it through the Targeted Keto Diet or the Cyclical Keto Diet.

You might encounter some people who argue that performance is affected while you are on a Ketogenic diet. This is not entirely true. There was a study performed on trained cyclists undergoing the Ketogenic Diet. The results showed that their aerobic endurance remained good and was not affected at all. Also, their muscle mass remained the same as it had been when they had started. The cyclists' bodies adapted to the diet through ketosis, and their bodies limited glycogen and glucose storage and utilized fats for converting into energy.

During the time of the research, this group of cyclists was fed on a rigorous diet of proteins, green vegetables, and a good quantity of fats. Thus, even when you do more cardio exercises, the Ketogenic Diet helps you a lot.

The only time when ketosis can make you suffer in performance is when you need give explosive performance. When you need some boost in your workouts, you may take in more carbohydrates by consuming 25-30 grams of the same approximately 30 minutes prior to your training.

Hazards of a ketogenic diet:

You will probably find many people trying to scare you away from a low carbohydrate diet. But don't worry; they're likely under some misconceptions which are more famous than the Keto Diet itself. There have been hundreds of studies conducted with people who have followed the Keto Diet. The studies and research have proved that fewer carbohydrates and more fats are beneficial for health. Strangely, people confuse the Ketogenic diet with a high carbs and high fats diet- a combination which is dreadful for the body. Obviously, when you eat tremendous amounts of food rich in fats as well as sugars, you are heading towards trouble.

If you have been thinking about going on a low fat diet, please think again. The Ketogenic Diet has been proven to be more effective for losing weight than a low fat diet. If you consume foods rich in carbohydrate content, your body produces glucose naturally. As we have already mentioned, our body finds it easiest to process carbohydrates and therefore, the body will look for them first. This results in immediate storage of excess fat in different parts of the body. This makes you gain weight and also gifts you with other ailments correlated with a high carbs-high fat diet, but not with the Ketogenic Diet.

Just to be safe, please check with a physician if you have any doubts about starting the Ketogenic Diet. You will also need to take precautions if you have a family history of diabetes or kidney ailments, because if you take in more proteins, it will put more strain on the kidneys.

High blood sugar, heart disease and high cholesterol are not the things you need to be concerned about. A high fat, low carbs diet is documented and known for improving blood sugar, cholesterol and reducing heart risks in your body.

What changes does your body undergo during the Ketogenic Diet?

Our bodies are adapted to the simplest routine of processing carbohydrates and utilizing them as energy. As a result, the body has an army of enzymes which are used in this metabolism, while it has only a small amount of enzymes which process fats. Even the enzymes which process the fats, mostly have the job of storing them. When our bodies suddenly have to adapt to a shortage of glucose and high levels of fats, it is a lot of work for our bodies. They have to build a new army of enzymes adaptive to process fats. However, God has gifted us with amazing bodies which can do wonders when called on to adapt to any situation.

When our bodies are pushed into a state of ketosis, they naturally use what is remaining of the glucose. This implies that our bodies will exhaust up all the glycogen from our muscles, which can temporarily cause weakness or a feeling of low energy. You might feel lethargic for a few days. In the initial few weeks, you may experience mental fogginess, headaches, symptoms of flu (also called Keto-flu), irritability, and dizziness. Some people also called it a PMS for all!

Usually, these sicknesses are a result of your body flushing out electrolytes. Therefore, you may also pass more urine in the initial days of the Ketogenic Diet. You must ensure that you keep up your intake of sodium, and drink plenty of water. You can increase your salt consumption to large amounts. Take salt with everything possible. Doesn't that sound good? You do not have to keep any check on your salt intake. Salt helps your body to retain water and also helps to replenish electrolytes.

The average person who begins the Ketogenic Diet will take approximately 2 weeks to cut down his carbohydrate intake to 25-40 grams. However, it is best if you can cut down the carb intake to as low as 15 grams so that you can get on the right track in just one week. Therefore, the less time you take to reach the state of ketosis, the less time you will have to bear the feeling of sickness.

If you are a regular gym goer, you may notice that you may lose a little endurance and strength at first. As already mentioned, this is normal for everyone. However, you will soon reach sustainable levels of energy throughout the day.

Chapter 4

What, apart from willpower, is needed to start the Ketogenic Diet?

How to get started

When you eat fat rich foods, consume moderate amounts of proteins and few carbs, it has a massive effect on your health. You are already aware of the benefits of the Ketogenic Diet, despite its initial side effects. In the initial weeks, you might crave carbohydrates, but that phase will pass gradually. Artificial sweeteners are linked with sugar cravings. Thus, if you usually consume diet sodas or artificial sweeteners, you will need to flush them out of your system. Having a strong willpower and the right diet chart will help you transform your eating philosophies.

Did you cheat on your diet chart?

Hmm… So, you have finally cheated on your Keto Diet. It's okay once in a while. But ideally, this should not go on forever. If you have been off the track for a few days, you will definitely want to get back to your healthy Keto regime as soon as possible. Obviously, it feels good when you know that you are healthy from the inside.

It sounds simple, but sometimes it can be a monumental challenge. Once you cheat just for a non-Keto meal, you feel dreadful the next morning. You might feel bloated, shaky, and exhausted. Yes, it happens. Remember, when you switched to the Keto Diet, you felt the same sickness. Now when your body has adapted to the Ketogenic Diet, it will definitely shake when it does not get its regular diet of fats.

So, now you know that since you have cheated once, you might do it again. Thus, it is better to be prepared for the next time. Take a look at the following tips and note down whichever you find appropriate for you.

1. **Whatever you like to do, do not beat yourself up**

This is the most important advice given to ketogenic followers. There is a large group of ketogenic disciples who blame themselves for not having enough willpower to manage their new diet. Well, you are a human being and all of us fail sometimes. There is nothing to blame yourself about. We live in a world full of gluten and sugar. We have to face the temptation daily at some place or the other. If you do not give in to these temptations even 80% of times, you are a winner. It is an achievement to have even this much willpower.
Suppose your friend cheated once on their diet. Would you beat them? Never... So why do you do it to yourself? Just keep on trying!

2. **Be responsible for your behavior**

Do not take the first tip as an excuse. If you ate a bowlful of ice-cream at the party last night, take responsibility for it. If your body feels awful after cheating, positively take responsibility for it. Make a note of situations when you are tempted to cheat. For example, when you leave home for the office, do not forget to take some fat bombs along. If you are tempted to eat due to emotions, or due to boredom, or for some other reason, note down such situations and be prepared for them in advance. Don't allow yourself to become too hungry- when you are already full, you will be less likely to stuff yourself more.

3. **Either have a salad for breakfast or do not have breakfast after a night of cheating**

After you have cheated on the Keto Diet, you must take a strictly Keto meal after that. If you had a non-Keto meal at night, you might even like to skip your breakfast the next day. Intermittent fasting has been recognized as a healthy practice worldwide. You can eat later when you truly feel hungry. Do not eat just for the sake of eating. Eat when your body demands it. You will not feel weak at all.
Also, eating a plate full of Keto vegetables is just like healing your stomach after you have had an unhealthy meal. But, eat it only if you feel like eating. You will feel rejuvenated.

4. Make notes

Remember the good old school days when you used to make notes for every important thing so that you could cram them for exams? Similarly, you just need to note down the good as well as bad feelings you have towards your ketogenic regime. Fix a day in the week to write down your feelings briefly.

If you felt good for several weeks, write it down. If you felt awful after a meal of cheating, then write it down immediately. It is easy to forget your bad feelings once you overcome the inflammation, headaches and stomachaches. This simple practice of writing will give you a much more real and objective picture of your diet.

5. Go get moving

When you run or take a brisk walk for a few kilometers to get rid of the hangover after too much to drink, it helps your body break down all the harmful material you dumped into it the previous night. The same process works for food hangovers too. When you have a heavy, unhealthy meal, make sure that you make some time to work out. It does not have to be a vigorous workout, but should at least raise your heart rate a little and work out your bowels. You will definitely feel better once you make this a habit.

6. Cut down on alcohol

There is no doubt that alcohol is a toxic substance, even if it is just wine. When you take in alcohol, especially hard drinks, you have a high chance of losing your willpower and cheating on your meals. Thus, it is better to have as little alcohol as you can. Moreover, if you do take it, make sure that you digest it properly and get rid of the hangover.

7. Sip low carb liquids and lots of water frequently

It is advice given regularly by all dieticians, but it needs to be repeated often. We cannot emphasize this fact enough that you can flush out all the unhealthy molecules in your body by drinking appropriate amounts of water. If you are prone to boredom eating and feel like you want to stuff your mouth with something every hour, then you should rather choose warm water or flavored cold water over snacks. Look for your favorite flavors of herbal tea without sweeteners.

If you need something more satisfying, you can try sipping some warm bone broth. This will fill you up without adding any extra carbs to your diet. You can also add some turmeric to the bone broth to add flavor and take advantage of its anti-inflammatory properties.

8. Do not leave home hungry

When you leave home, make sure that you eat something healthy first. When you leave on an empty stomach, you will be more tempted to grab a burger or other fast food. You succumb to your temptations more easily when you are hungry. When you do not feel hungry, you have 90% less chance of cheating on Keto.

9. Do not punish or deprive yourself

Do not go overboard with the Ketogenic Diet and become a maniac. Just because you have started a healthy diet does not mean that you cannot eat when you want to. As already mentioned, if you are prone to boredom eating or emotional eating, keep some healthy substitutes with you. If you feel hungry, then please eat. Eating only a plate of salad a day for weeks at a time is not a good idea at all. These kinds of habits eventually make you even more prone to giving in to your temptations.

10. Find a support group or a buddy

There are many benefits to doing the Keto Diet with friends or with a support group. You get the required emotional support and you become accountable to someone. It is sometimes really difficult to keep promises to yourself. When you make a promise to your conscience, it is much easier to pretend that you never made it and you can just break it anytime. When you declare it to someone else, you feel more strongly that you have to abide by it.

If you cannot find any real friends to support you, you can join any online forum. Such virtual support is also helpful, because obviously real people are there on the other end. You can also get some amazingly easy recipes from these forums.

11. Develop cooking as a hobby

If you have been shying away from cooking throughout your life, now is the right time to pick the hobby up. When you cook something amazing, you feel encouraged to try and cook even more. Motivate yourself and look for some easy and fun recipes to support your Ketogenic Diet.

Chapter 5

What are the common mistakes committed by Keto followers? As we have already mentioned before, if you have any doubts about the Ketogenic Diet, you must consult your physician. This high fat and low carb diet does not suit everyone. Though you probably know all the benefits of the Ketogenic diet, you also need to know where you can go wrong. Ketones are really beneficial as a fuel for the diaphragm and the heart. The state of ketosis can provide you with great cognitive performance and a good amount of focus. If you are an endurance athlete, this diet can prove extremely beneficial for distance swimming, cycling, ultra-running, or marathons.

However, there are not many resources available around us that can lead us to ketosis without experiencing nutrition deficiency if your Ketogenic diet goes wrong. Moreover, these deficiencies can get really big if you work out a lot. In addition, consuming MCT oil and coconut oil can get really, really boring very soon.

So, you must be thinking, "If there are so many stumbling blocks in my way to reaching the state of ketosis, is this diet worth the effort?" Yes, it is, definitely. It is not as difficult as it sounds. But it is crucial to have a basic understanding of the metabolism of your body and its nutritional needs before your march ahead with this diet plan.

You must also find out about the common mistakes committed by people who are already following this diet. Prepare yourself with a lot of ketogenic recipes and then go ahead and begin your new lifestyle.

Mistake No.1   Being afraid of fat

Obviously you know that you need to consume more fats than ever in the Ketogenic Diet. But the fact is that most of us are not able to overcome the mental block of thinking of fats as evil. The food industry has brainwashed us for many decades that we need to consume as few fats as we can in order to remain healthy. But the fact is that even on a non-Keto diet, we must consume some amount of fats to remain healthy. Even more in the Ketogenic Diet, where we have to derive our energy from fatty acids instead of glucose, we have to consume even more fats without any guilt. Since we are not consuming many carbohydrates, we must not shy away from fats. Eat full fat cheese, eat the skin of the chicken, soak the broccoli in butter…. yeah… you are right. You have to eat as much fat as you can. The only fats you need to keep away from are vegetable oils like corn and canola. Such oils do not help cure inflammation in our bodies.

Even when you see that you need to consume massive amounts of meat and oils, try to remember that fat is not "evil" for your body. But do consume fats under the right guidance. You would not like to end up getting sick.

Mistake No.2   Consuming an excess of protein

Beginners of the Ketogenic Diet make another common blunder of replacing carbohydrates with proteins. This can lead you to gluconeogenesis, which means that amino acids are converted to glucose. But this is the exact opposite of what we need on a Ketogenic diet. We need to keep the glucose levels at a lower level and speed up the process of making ketones from fatty acids.

The fact is that you actually need to consume very small amounts of protein because fats are protein sparing. That means that our bodies' requirement of protein goes down with the high intake of fats. Thus, you do not need to worry if you are consuming fewer carbs. Do not try to compensate for them with proteins.

Mistake No. 3   Quitting too early

When you enter into the state of ketosis quickly, you might initially suffer from side effects. The changes in metabolism can be really dramatic because every cell of your body has to switch from the metabolism of glucose to fats. Your insulin levels go down due to lower levels of carbohydrates. This also affects your kidneys, which adapt to hold on to the sodium available in the body. When the insulin level is consistently low, the kidneys also shed sodium and water.

This is why it is always recommended that you consume more sodium and drink plenty of water, particularly in the initial phase. It helps to escape the Keto-flu. It is more appropriate if we call the symptoms "symptoms of carbohydrate withdrawal" due to the effect on electrolyte and hormonal balance.

These facts might seem intimidating to you. But you must pledge to yourself that you will not quit regardless of a little sickness in the initial days. You can consume strong bone broth containing high quality salt. You must also take a lot of rest and not work out intensely. Also, drink lots of water rich in minerals.

Moreover, the best advice is that you must go slowly when you begin the Ketogenic Diet. Do not give up when you feel sick during the first couple of weeks, and make sure you get all the recommended blood tests done. This will ensure that your body is not suppressing any health issues that do not appear on the surface.

Mistake No.4   Carbohydrates creep in

It sounds very obvious. But, it is not very simple as it sounds. Carbohydrates can seep in even from those sources which you think are carb-free. If you are fond of buying herbs, spices and vegetables, you might experience an increase in your carbs intake. Some products that you buy from the market with all the best intentions may contain carbs. For instance, factory made salad dressing, tomato sauces, substitutes for milk like almond milk and coconut milk have sugar added in them, meats such as duck meat, starchy vegetables, some kinds of herbal tea- these are just a few products which might contain carbohydrates.

It might become a challenge for you to eat out because many bars and restaurants use dressings, dips and sauces, which have additional sugar or honey. It definitely tastes good but is not good for your diet at all.

You must have solid, dependable information for restricting your carbohydrates intake, particularly in the initial phase when your body undergoes drastic changes.

Mistake No.5   Munching processed foods

This mistake is commonly committed by people who have read the Atkins diet (a low carb diet), and observed the foods which are sold online. No doubt that these foods keep your body at low carbohydrate levels and make your life a lot simpler. But the equally true fact is that these foods have high contents of artificial flavors, coloring, sucralose, polydextrose, and many other artificial sweeteners. These things obviously play havoc with your mental and physical health.

You might feel that you are not familiar with half of the ingredients mentioned in the Keto diet list or you are not aware of the shops which supply them. Do yourself a favor and make an effort find them out. The rule of thumb of the Ketogenic Diet is that if you are not able to cook or bake a meal out of these ingredients, then you must keep away from them.

The time is not far away when most of the food companies will start manufacturing foods made out of real ingredients because the trend of being concerned about one's health is reaching its peak really fast. So, be patient and be the pioneer of the Ketogenic Diet among your friends. They should also feel motivated when they see your dedication.

Mistake No.6 Eating the same recipes time and again and panicking when faced with new recipes

In the initial phase, when you feel overwhelmed by eating low carbs foods, you might always want to eat the same "safe" line of foods habitually. This is because you do not have much knowledge and experience of ketogenic recipes. That is why it is always recommended that you prepare yourself with a lot of ketogenic recipes before you start.

Suppose you had to eat eggs and bacon for every breakfast and nuts for snacks all the time. Wouldn't you get bored in just a couple of days? This is really common with most Keto practitioners. Even if you are not a Keto follower, you cannot eat the same pizza for breakfast, lunch and dinner over and over again!

Even when you eat low carb foods in your new regime, you must focus on improving your health. This is possible only with a varied and nutritious diet. Every individual is different. If your Keto friend loves bacon for breakfast, you might not like it.

Eat what you love and keep changing your routine. The same routine causes boredom to set in. That's not the only problem, though. Eating the same foods over and over may also cause nutritional deficiencies in your body and you may even become intolerant towards some foods. This would happen especially if you are very stressed or if you are on any kind of medication.

Intolerance for food sets off cramps, bloating, constipation, diarrhea, and many other symptoms. This not only impacts the gut health but also your immune system. The best thing is to keep trying new Keto-friendly foods, even if you have not ever heard of them. For example, chicken liver is a relatively unfamiliar thing for most people. But it's easy to find and to prepare. The long list of Keto-friendly foods can be transformed into many delicious recipes. So don't just stick to a couple of recipes you know. That will make you quit even faster.

Mistake No.7 A lack of planning

One of the major stumbling blocks on the Ketogenic Diet is a lack of planning. If you do not plan well, there is a good chance that you will fail. For example, you are already aware that your kitchen should be well stocked with most of the Keto-friendly ingredients. But what happens when one day you realize that you do not have enough coconut milk in your fridge? You might panic and get frustrated because the shop near the corner street does not sell coconut milk. Many Keto ingredients which are staples for a low carb diet such as oily fish, olives, coconut oil, ghee, etc. are available only online or in health shops. More supermarkets are coming up with ketogenic products nowadays. Still, you need to plan properly and be well aware that you would need these products. Thus, when you visit the shop next time that stocks Keto goods, you must buy more than you need for just a meal. You can also cook ketogenic recipes in bulk and save on your time as well as money.

Mistake No.8   Getting too obsessed with the diet

Another major obstacle in the Ketogenic diet is being too obsessed with the diet. You might love to plan every last bite of the day in the initial stages. However, this is not practicable. It is feasible though for those patients who have been recommended the Ketogenic Diet due to any medication or sickness like epilepsy. In such ailments, every bite has to be planned without any chance of failure. Otherwise the patient might have to face serious consequences.

However, since you have chosen the Ketogenic Diet yourself, you must not get too stressed over your dietary changes. The new routine should not interfere with your mental balance. Do not become a maniac thinking what your next meal should be or how you can increase your ketones or what you should eat on the vacation next weekend!

In order to avoid such craziness, you should sometimes just relax and make a few recipes without counting and weighing. You can also give yourself some more time if you feel so and do not feel guilty about it. If you remain under mental stress about your food, you will not be able to enjoy the physical benefits of the Ketogenic Diet. Physical benefits take even more time to show up when you have mental turmoil going on.

Mistake No.9   Ignoring the warning signs of your body

People who get obsessed with the changes in their diets can end up measuring ketones and blood glucose in their body and weighing the food every time, making exact plans for meals, etc. They are even literally scared of eating at restaurants where they cannot actually control their food. According to the experts, these people are the ones who mostly ignore the warning signs given by their body. For example, perhaps you know that there is a particular ketogenic recipe that you do not like and your tummy feels bloated when you eat it. Still, you eat it because you "know" that it is good for your body. As a matter of fact, your body knows better than you do. Do not ignore the signs given by your body. If a food does not make you feel good from inside, then do not eat it.

In another instance, at some stage you might not feel like exerting your body to do high intensity training. If you go ahead just because it was on the chart for the day, you might end up hurting your ligaments.

No meal or training or expert advice can take over your innate intuition and knowledge. Do take the warning signs seriously and do not foolishly stick to your regime even when your body is telling you not to do so.

The Ketogenic Diet or other low carb diets are not suitable for everyone. If you do not feel better than before you switched to the Ketogenic Diet (after the initial phase of sickness, of course) you might like to reconsider your decision.

Mistake No.10   Giving in to social pressure

Our social lives are a big factor which should never underestimate. Even if our friends and family do not mean to pull us back from our healthy regime; they probably will not stop teasing us. We have to listen to comments like, "Oh, come on dear, you are here to party! Don't be a spoil sport. You will not die if you eat just one slice of pizza!" And so we give in.

It is of course impossible to try and explain about the Ketogenic Diet and its benefits every time. Nobody wants to listen to your blabbing and of course, you would also not like to show off your new lifestyle all the time. Although your family knows about the benefits you have experienced from the Ketogenic Diet, they probably still won't stop pushing you to have another piece of cake.

Furthermore, many medical professionals do not understand the true concept of the Ketogenic Diet. However, it is a well-established fact that you can go by the 80/20 rule, and this allows you to have some breaks and enjoy a few treats in moderate amounts. But, when you are completely in ketosis, you will probably find that you truly do not feel like eating anything apart from the stipulated foods. They actually do not make you feel good when you are in ketosis. When you eat a slice of cake during this state, it actually does not feel good.

- **Mistake No.11   Poor timing**

Another crucial factor in determining the success of the Ketogenic Diet is the timing when you start it. You must consider the circumstances that are present when you are about to start this diet. Since the Ketogenic Diet demands a lot of attention, care and rest; you must not start at least a week before something important is expected. For example, if you have a very important meeting in your office next week, do not start it now.

Also, if you are going through a busy season professionally, you must not start this diet. You can begin this regime when you have ample time in hand to rest if you feel frail in the initial phase of keto. When off season times are going on in your profession, then you can think about starting it. This would allow you to take rest or even a holiday if you cannot work at all.

Mistake No.12   Not providing enough time for the body to transition

In the initial week, your bowel habits may change. You may experience constipation or diarrhea, but it will regulate over time. For some people, fiber supplements help in curing stomach problems. But, for others, fiber may not help at all. Thus, you may want to seek personal advice from your physician before eating lots of fiber.

The adaptation may even take up to a month. Many people also experience an energy blast, euphoric feelings, along with a lot of fat loss. Your urine may smell strange and you might also develop some kind of metallic taste in the mouth. However, you do not have to be worried. These changes are a sign that your new diet is working.

Mistake No. 13   Testing ketosis with urine ketone testing sticks

This is a big mistake some people make. Low carbohydrate diet followers have relied on the urine ketone testing sticks for a very long time. These sticks test the level of acetoacetate your boy is excreting. You may find it extremely thrilling to see the sticks turn dark purple from light pink. It makes you feel good about your body, but unfortunately, these sticks do not show exact results. Moreover, they cannot show the particular type of ketones your body uses as a fuel.

A more accurate test is the blood test for checking beta-hydroxybutyrate. It will give you a better picture of whether you are adapted to keto or not, or if your body is burning ketones and fat for fuel- which is the actual essence of the Ketogenic Diet.

The information you gain about blood ketones rather than urine ketones is absolute gold regarding your performance on your low carbohydrate diet.

Mistake No. 14   Eating too much or too often

It is very common in our society to eat by the clock and to eat much more than it is required to feed our stomachs. You have probably been doing this on your high-carb diet. But it is a blunder if you do the same with your ketogenic diet. When you eat a high fat and low carb diet, your body really does not require food for many hours in a row. So do not feel worried about it. People often indulge in three full meals in a day along with snacks. Trust the experts' advice, they would never recommend that you eat this much every day.

Your body can eat up the fats it has stored for energy and sustain effectively. You would not feel deprived even if you do not eat. You have to eat food only when you feel hungry.

Mistake No. 15   Falling short of maintaining blood sugar levels

You must be thinking, "Why do I have to measure my blood sugar when I am not a diabetic?" The fact is that every one of us should keep a check on it. When your blood sugar is normalized during ketosis, it keeps your hunger down, regulates your mood and gives you a sense of well-being. Moreover, when your blood sugar is regulated, it is easier to attain nutritional ketosis and vice versa.

Chapter 6

How can you avoid Ketogenic Diet mistakes?

By now, you must have got an idea that you need tons of patience and perseverance to stay healthy with the Ketogenic Diet. Besides this, you also need a few tricks and tips mentioned in the previous chapters to stick to this new lifestyle. It is easy to give in to social pressure and your own temptations, but you have to be determined and convince your friends and family that this is not just a new fad and that you truly want to transform your body for good.

This can happen only when you are yourself convinced that you have chosen the right track. When your family members see the changes in your body and your health, they might also get motivated to adapt this way of eating.

You have already read the common mistakes people commit. To avoid these pitfalls, you must keep the points listed below in mind. Even if you find them repetitive, they have been mentioned to stress the facts you need to remember at all times.

1. Give yourself enough time to adapt

Never ever start the Ketogenic Diet if you do not have enough time to give to your body for adaptation. You must have at least a couple of weeks in hand to overcome the keto fever and other symptoms like constipation and diarrhea. It's probably best not to start this routine just a week before your holiday. It might spoil your holiday mood and make you feel low.

Such things discourage you a lot and get you off the track sooner than ever. You must be motivated enough to keep up with anything new that you pick up.

2. Ask for support from your friends and family

Since you may also experience mood swings due to the drastic changes in your diet, you may want to inform some of your loved ones about your new routine and ask for their cooperation and support.

Your true well-wishers will be more than happy to help you in this important step of your life. You can also ask them to prohibit you from indulging in non-keto food even when you feel tempted to do so.

They may tease you at times, but do not feel disheartened. Be brave and take it in good spirits. When you give cheerful replies to people, they are even happier with you. When you are in a bad mood, alert them of the situation and tell them to beware of you! You would not like to spoil your relationships forever just because of a couple of hours of mood swings. When you take proper precautionary steps without worrying too much, you are bound to succeed.

3. Stay around motivating factors

You must make friends with people who are positive in their lives and do not pull you down all the time. If you stay around negative people, they might turn out to not be your well-wishers. They are not happy to see anyone succeed and will be happy if you fail.

On the other hand, positive people themselves want to succeed in the smallest things in their lives and are happy to see others do so. They encourage you to keep trying even after you fall at times. They will encourage you to rise up and double your efforts. Spend time with both types of people for one week in your life before starting this routine and you will definitely see the difference the two groups make to your outlook.

4. Keep visiting the physician

Do not ignore this piece of advice. You might think that you have read enough and gained much knowledge from people around you, but it is always advisable to seek the advice of a physician you trust. It is worth spending the money in advance rather than thinking of saving it. If you end up making any major mistakes in the Ketogenic Diet, you may have to face some serious consequences and pay much more money than you should have.

Also, it is important to visit a trustworthy physician. He must be able to diagnose you properly and give required advice. There are some physicians who deliberately give you the wrong advice so that you fail frequently and visit them more often so that they can make more money. Beware of such doctors.

If you do not have a family physician in your vicinity, ask your friends who have been following the Ketogenic Diet lately. By all means, get help from internet forums, but please also follow the advice of your doctor.

5. Do not go maniac

Yes, you have taken a major step in your life, but nobody would like to see you going nuts over this new ketogenic diet. This fact cannot be stressed enough that we advocate this diet only to see you healthier, and not to see you getting obsessed with ketones and ketosis. You need to make peace with your eating habits. If you do not feel motivated enough to follow this regime, think again if you really want to do it for the rest of your life.

Your body must feel good after making so much effort. If this is not the case, you must seek the advice of your friends and family who have the know-how of the Ketogenic Diet. They might enlighten you if you are not able to decide. But do give yourself ample time to adjust before you want to re-think.

It is always easy to step back once you have decided to do something, but it is not so easy to get back to the same milestone once you have crossed it.

6. Keep yourself well equipped

As you must have already read, keep your kitchen well stocked in advance so that you do not fall short of supplies when you need to cook anything. Since this diet is almost entirely based on fats, it might prove a little expensive for you. Thus, it is better to buy things in larger quantities to save money. Groceries always prove cheaper when bought in bigger packets and of course, they last much longer. Find stores online which keep groceries specifically for the Ketogenic Diet. You'll probably get your stuff from such stores at much cheaper rates than you would at the local supermarket. Such stores cater to the needs of the Ketogenic Diet followers and stock products required by them. They also procure the groceries at cheaper prices and hence supply them to you at comparatively competitive rates. An occasional supplier of ketogenic supplies will charge much higher than the things are worth. Hence, make an effort and find out places that suit you and your budget.

When you keep the pitfalls and precautionary measures in mind, you will be less likely to fail. It is always better to be well prepared rather than repent later. Keep on the right track and you will definitely reap the fruits soon.

Conclusion

After reading this entire book on the Ketogenic Diet: *Ketogenic Diet Mistakes You Need to Know*, you must be feeling more at ease. It is always good to hear from a reliable source about an important thing that you have been anxious about. The Ketogenic Diet is not at all mysterious in itself but people who have not succeeded in it, have made it so. They have spread such myths about the Ketogenic Diet that even those who have the guts to start it, have to think twice before doing it.

All of us have at least enough willpower to take any new step. The rest of the journey is covered with the help of new milestones and support from our family and friends. You do not need to panic about this diet. Every single human being among us is capable of achieving much more they can imagine. Even the biggest deeds of the world were started as baby steps towards achieving something new. Perseverance and good intentions lead people to achieve what they have always wanted.

Have you ever read the autobiography of an athlete or an Olympic winner? Most of them come from humble backgrounds. They just have big dreams. In the initial stages of their career, even they are doubtful about their success, but as the time passes and they stay patient and keep up the hard work, all their efforts pay off well.

Similarly, even if you are an ordinary person with no Olympic aspirations, you cannot underestimate your determination and your motivation. All of us want to have a healthy body and remain disease free throughout our lives. But only a few of us are able to achieve it. It's not that those who have been successful in achieving the state of ketosis have not faced any obstacles. It is just a matter of facing these troubles bravely and overcoming your temptations. The victorious keto-followers have resisted their temptations well. Eventually, when you are able to say, "No, thank you" to mouthwatering cuisines for quite some time, you even start disliking that type of food.

Thus, just keep your eyes on the end results that you are going to have a good body once you have your ketones working for you instead of carbohydrates. I'm sure you will be able to make an effort with even more dedication than you think. Good luck with this life transforming ketogenic diet!

www.ingramcontent.com/pod-product-compliance
Lightning Source LLC
LaVergne TN
LVHW010439070526
838199LV00066B/6092